SHIATSU THERAPY

For Further Reference;
SHIATSU: Japanese Finger-Pressure Therapy
by Tokujiro Namikoshi
84 pp., 7½ × 10½ in., 100 black-and-white photos,
paperback, LC-68-19983, ISBN 0-87040-169-6

SHIATSU: Health and Vitality at Your Fingertips
by Tokujiro Namikoshi
84 pp., 7½ × 10½ in., 100 black-and-white photo,
hard-cover, LC-68-19983, ISBN 0-87040-115-7

SHIATSU THERAPY
Theory and Practice

By Toru Namikoshi

JAPAN PUBLICATIONS, INC.

Published by
JAPAN PUBLICATIONS, INC., Tokyo, Japan
Distributed by
JAPAN PUBLICATIONS TRADING COMPANY
1255 Howard Street, San Francisco, California 94103, U. S. A.
P. O. Box 5030 Tokyo International, Tokyo 101-31, Japan

First edition: July 1974

LCC Card No. 74-79314
ISBN 0-87040-270-6

Printed in Japan

Preface

The first goal of shiatsu is to apply a distinctive kind of pressure therapy to relieve fatigue, generate pleasant sensations, and thus stimulate the body to use its innate, natural powers of recuperation. For shiatsu purposes, there are a number of points on the surface of the body where pressure applications produce remarkable results. These points are located at important places over muscles, bones, nerves, blood vessels, lymph vessels, and glands of the endocrine system. The kind of pressure applied, the way it is applied, and the proper pressure points on the body depend on the nature of the patient's complaint.

Pollution is a problem of immense importance in the modern world. The natural environment is being violated, and man is being submitted to dangerous influences and all kinds of harmful substances. Even medicines, which are designed to be of benefit, often have side effects that are extremely harmful. Shiatsu helps the body recover its own strength and involves nothing that can have any unpleasant or harmful side effects. In this respect, shiatsu is a therapeutic system in complete accord with nature.

The popularity and fame of shiatsu, originally a Japanese therapeutic system, have reached all parts of the world. This is a source of great joy for me. I am trying to do as much as I can to spread more accurate knowledge about the nature of shiatsu and the benefits it can bring. To that end I have written this book. I intend to exert maximum effort toward inspiring people in education, medicine, sports, cosmetics, health, welfare, and all other fields to take advantage of what shiatsu can offer. If this book and its companion volume, *Shiatsu: Health and Vitality at your Fingertips*, by Tokujiro Namikoshi, president of the Nippon Shiatsu School, can bring even one more person to an understanding of shiatsu, I shall be very happy.

TORU NAMIKOSHI

Contents

Chapter 1 | The Theory of Shiatsu Therapy

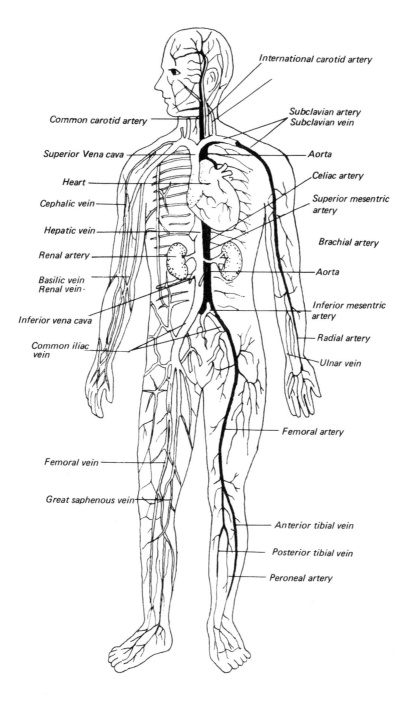

International carotid artery

Common carotid artery

Subclavian artery
Subclavian vein

Superior Vena cava

Aorta

Heart

Celiac artery

Cephalic vein

Superior mesentric artery

Hepatic vein

Brachial artery

Renal artery

Aorta

Basilic vein
Renal vein

Inferior mesentric artery

Inferior vena cava

Radial artery

Common iliac vein

Ulnar vein

Femoral artery

Femoral vein

Great saphenous vein

Anterior tibial vein

Posterior tibial vein

Peroneal artery

What Is Shiatsu Therapy?

Fundamentally shiatsu is quite simple. It relies on the proper application of carefully judged pressures on specific points on the surfaces of the human body to eliminate fatigue and stimulate the body's natural self-curative abilities. This pressure is applied with the fingers and hands. The Japanese word *shiatsu* is composed of a character meaning finger (*shi*) and another character meaning pressure (*atsu*).

A kind of shiatsu has probably been practiced by human beings since the very dawn of humanity itself. When a part of the body is sluggish or in pain, the natural reaction is to press or rub it with the hands. This reaction is probably the true origin of shiatsu therapy. But over many years of diligent study and research, such instinctive treatment has been scientifically systematized and improved to become a therapeutic method adjusted to the demands of a variety of ailments.

But shiatsu is not strictly speaking medicine; it is primarily a way to prevent the development of sickness and a therapy ideally suited to human instincts. Unfortunately, modern medicine, based almost entirely on medical and surgical treatment, has reached an impasse because it has overlooked the natural curative powers of the body. Medical science has tended to have a weakening effect on the human body's natural resistance and to devote attention solely to coping with symptoms once illness has appeared. Consequently, patients sometimes reach such poor physical condition that the best skills of doctors are unable to effect cures. Shiatsu is based on the opposite approach: it strives always to keep the body in top condition so that symptoms requiring medical attention do not develop.

Shiatsu was originally a purely Japanese treatment system, but today it is steadily growing popular in many parts of the world. The Namikoshi Institute of Shiatsu Therapy was the first of its kind. In 1940, it was the only institution devoted solely to shiatsu in Japan, In 1955, the Japanese Ministry of Health and Welfare recognized shiatsu as a valid treatment in a general category with traditional Japanese massage (*amma*) and Western-style massage. Since that time, the Nippon Shiatsu School has continued to expand and develop. The Namikoshi shiatsu system is the only pure and correct shiatsu system.

Characteristics of Shiatsu Therapy

1. Immediate diagnosis

As he presses from place to place over the body, the shiatsu practitioner is immediately able to diagnose the patient's condition and determine the specific kind of therapy needed. The skilled shiatsu technician has developed a sense of touch that enables him to spot irregularities in blood circulation, lymph stagnation, abnormal internal secretions, deformitites in the skeleton, and undue pressures exerted on the nerves. He will examine the skin to see whether it is rough or smooth, hot, or cold. The information he derives from this examination and from an estimation of the conditions of the muscles enables him to diagnose the cause of the trouble and to know what treatment to use.

2. No medicines or mechanical devices needed

Shiatsu can be performed anywhere and at any time since it employs nothing but the human hands.

3. No unpleasant sensations or secondary effects

Shiatsu therapy is pleasant and produces no unpleasant sensations or pains even in a patient whose muscles are stiff. Since no medicines, injections, or mechanical devices are used, shiatsu produces no unpleasant secondary effects. Its beneficial effects manifest themselves gradually.

4. Suitable to all age groups

In young children, shiatsu helps produce strong bodies and to ward off illness. It helps adults guard against sicknesses common to their age level, and it retards aging and helps ensure longevity and continued health and strength in the old.

5. Resistance to sickness

The person who undergoes shiatsu treatment learns to recognize the effects of fatigue and in this way develops a kind of health barometer within himself. Regular, periodic shiatsu therapy keeps the skin and muscles flexible and stimulates the regenerative powers of the cellular structures of the body and its organs. This has the effect of creating a self-defense mechanism that increases the body's powers of resistance and thus lowers the likelihood of sickness.

6. Sense of mutual trust and reliance

Ideally, shiatsu treatment is a relationship in which the patient and the practitioner exchange roles and in this way strengthen the effect of the treatment and stimulate a profound feeling of trust in the treatment and in each other.

The proper relation between the person administrating shiatsu treatment and the person receiving it is illustrated by the hen and chick. Before the eggs are ready to hatch, the hen broods on them. When the young chick inside the egg begins to stir, the hen senses what is about to happen and begins to peck gently, yet firmly, on the outside of the shell. The chick answers by pecking at the same place on the inside of the shell. The two working together break the shell, and a new life begins. In shiatsu too, the practitioner and the patient must work together to produce the desired effect of improved health and strength.

7. Total treatment

If shiatsu were applied only to the part of the body in pain, its effect would be only temporary. Shiatsu itself would then be no more than a treatment of symptoms. But shiatsu strives to generate strength and health in the entire body; consequently, it is applied to all of the body parts, with emphasis on places manifesting symptoms of pain or discomfort.

Why Shiatsu Cures

To recapitulate, shiatsu strives to cure ailments and prevent their recurrence and the development of other ailments. Pressure applied by the hands on certain points of the skin stimulates the body's natural recuperative powers and removes fatigue by causing the diffusion of the lactic acid and carbon dioxide that accumulate among the tissues to cause muscular stiffness and stagnation of the blood. These accumulations of fatigue-causing materials apply abnormal pressure on the nerves, blood, and lymph vessels. This causes irregular internal secretions and peculiarities in the skeletal system and internal organs. By diffusing fatigue-causing accumulations, shiatsu pressure restores flexibility to the muscle tissues and relieves pain-producing symptoms.

Throughout the body there is a large number of places closely related to the functioning of the body organs and vessels. Shiatsu treatment is concerned mainly with the 660 zones (*tsubo*) where blood vessels, lymph vessels, nerves, and the ductless glands of the endocrine system tend to concentrate or to branch. Although the *tsubo* are invisible on the skin, they are nonetheless of the greatest importance. Namikoshi shiatsu therapy has organized the *tsubo* in a system that is based on physiology and pathology. Simply pressing on the body and stimulating a response is not enough to bring about truly therapeutic effects. One must have a correct and accurate knowledge of the *tsubo* and must know how to vary pressure, pressing method, and pressing frequency.

Seven Effects

The following seven interrelated shiatsu effects stimulate the body to operate normally and help maintain good health.
1. Invigorating the skin
2. Stimulating the circulation of the body fluids
3. Promoting suppleness in the muscular tissues
4. Correcting faults in the skeletal system
5. Promoting harmonious functioning of the nervous system
6. Regulating the operation of the ductless endocrine glands
7. Stimulating the normal functioning of the internal organs

1. Invigorating the skin

The following are the major functions of the skin.
(1) Protection from bacterial invasion
(2) Transmission of sense information (heat, cold, touch) and consequent warning of imminent danger
(3) Maintaining body temperature equilibrium (through evaporation as sweat and through the storing of subcutaneous fat for the sake of warmth)
(4) Excretion of wastes (sweat and sebum)
(5) Protection from harmful rays in sunlight

(6) Storage of water and nourishment (in the form of water
      and fat)

The skin is made up of three layers: the epidermis, or outermost
layer; the dermis, or inner layer; and the subcutaneous tissue.
The cells of the epidermis are constantly growing, and dead cells
are given off in the form of dandruff and the scum that one finds
in one's bathwater. The epidermis contains the melanin that gives
skin its color. Sweat glands are present in the skin in all parts of
the body, though they are especially plentiful in the armpits, palms,
and soles of the feet. These glands transport waste materials from
the blood stream to the outside of the body. Wastes are found in
sebum and in sweat. The sebaceous glands, which secrete sebum,
are present in the parts of the skin containing hair follicles.
Shiatsu pressure stimulates the activity of the sebaceous glands and
keeps the skin soft and lustrous. It also helps provide hair follicles
with greater nourishment. This helps keep hair more lustrous and
prevents its falling out. Nerve endings are found in the subcutaneous
layer of the skin. These are especially numerous in the hairless
areas, like the fingertips, where there are important sensory vessels.
The skin secretes a hormonelike substance said to have a subtle
effect on the basic life powers. In summary, shiatsu, which is
applied directly to the skin, improves metabolism by invigorating
the capillary action in the blood vessels. It stimulates the
transportation of nourishment to the skin, increases the skin's
powers of resistance, and by promoting general well being preserves
youthfulness.

2. Stimulating the circulation of the body fluids

The body fluids—mainly blood and lymph—are supplied to all of
the body tissues at varying speeds. By means of the action of the
capillaries of the circulation system, these fluids take nourishment
to the body cells and remove waste products, carbon dioxide, water,
and metabolic byproducts. The heart is the pump that keeps the
blood flowing smoothly. The blood passes out of the heart to the
body through the arteries, moves to all parts of the body via the
smaller arteries, carries out its food-supply and waste-removal
processes by means of the millions of capillaries in the body, and
then returns to the heart by way of the veins. The blood is
reoxygenated when it passes through the lungs. Shiatsu helps

maintain regularity and smoothness in the blood circulation and prevents stagnation and congestion in the system.

3. Promoting suppleness in the muscular tissues

In daily living, excess effort and tensions often result in stiffness in the muscles of the shoulders, neck, and back and sluggishness in the legs. This stiffness applies undue pressure on the blood and lymph vessels and on the nerves, and this in turn produces pain and other unpleasant sensations. If this condition is allowed to continue, the capillaries will fail to nourish the cells properly, and muscular irregularities and chronic stiffness will develop. Applications of shiatsu pressure relieve the stiffness and help the muscles to return to normal condition by stimulating the circulation of blood and lymph and the proper functioning of the capillaries in nourishing cells and removing wastes. Especially complicated conditions can develop on both sides of the spinal column because in this region cordlike muscles overlap. Muscular cells may be divided into the following three major categories.

1. Striated muscles (voluntarily controlled muscles, also called skeletal muscles). Attached to the skeletal framework, these muscles support the body and control the motions of the limbs and the trunk. There are approximately 600 muscles in the body, accounting for about 45 percent of total body weight. Of these, roughly 400 are striated skeletal muscles.
2. Smooth muscles (involuntarily controlled muscles). These are found in the tissues of the internal organs and of the walls of blood vessels.
3. Cardiac muscles (involuntarily controlled). This muscle is striated but operates completely involuntarily.

The following kinds of abnormalities may occur in muscle tissue.

1. Painful arrested contraction.
2. Paralysis and powerlessness.
3. Rigidity, in spite of ability to tense. This is caused by irregularities in the skin and tendons.
4. Trembling paralysis; writer's cramp is an example of this condition.

Commonly experienced conditions resulting from these abnormalities include backaches, cramps, cricks, the so-called whiplash effect, twisted neck, and so on.

4. Correcting faults in the skeletal system

The skeletal system of the human body consists of 206 bones arranged in the following major groups: the skull, the spinal column, the thorax, the pelvis, and the four limbs. The bones themselves are a hard tissue containing living cells responsible for growth and repair. The inorganic parts of the bone are calcium and phosphorous, but bones include a gelatinous material as well. A membrane serves to protect the bone and to provide nourishment and sensation since it contains blood and lymph vessels and nerves. The bony material is arranged in a dense structure of many layers around the spongy marrow, in which red and white blood corpuscles are produced.

Building up of fatigue reduces the amount of nourishment that reaches the bones because it weakens the flow of the body fluids that transport food. This can cause the bones themselves to become so brittle that they break easily, or it can result in malformations of the skeleton. With proper shiatsu treatment such conditions can be corrected. Shiatsu treatment applied to children can ensure correct bone development and help ward off illnesses involving the bone tissue. For unknown reasons, at puberty, which is a period of especially rapid growth, girls often experience bending of the bones. Parents must observe their children's posture closely. At the first sign of an abnormality, steps must be taken. If the trouble is spotted early, shiatsu can correct skeletal irregularities in young people.

5. Promoting harmonious functioning of the nervous system

The nervous system, which controls all bodily actions and operation, is divided into two major systems.
1. Brain and spinal cord
   These organs control conscious actions of the skeleton as well as perception through the skin and mucous membranes and all mental and psychological activity.
2. Autonomic nervous system
   This system is composed of the sympathetic and parasympathetic subsystems. It controls the involuntary functioning of the heart, stomach, intestines, reproductive organs, and endocrine glands. The sympathetic subsystem stimulates the activities of these organs, and the parasympathetic subsystem regulates

them. Shiatsu treatment can prevent nervous irregularities, especially in the vagus nerve, and can contribute to the smooth transmission of nervous impulses.

Applied to the head, shiatsu pressure stimulates the cerebral membrane and the pituitary gland, which regulate the motor nerves and the nerves controlling memory and commands to and from the brain. Shiatsu pressure on the front of the neck stimulates action of the vagus nerve and reactions in the arteries in the neck. This in turn helps control blood pressure and the operation of the heart and other internal organs. Shiatsu on the region of the afterbrain stimulates the pituitary gland and the nerves controlling the respiratory system. Pressure applied with the palms to the eyes stimulates the ends of the trigeminal nerves and the central spinal cord. It further stimulates the vagus nerve and helps control the heart.

Applied to the shoulder blades, shiatsu pressure affects the nerve plexuses in the arms and the sympathetic system controlling the internal organs.

Irregularities in the internal organs reflect in the sympathetic nervous system by causing agitation and the appearance of lumps or either side of the spinal column. Gentle shiatsu pressure on the back can relieve this condition. The Namikoshi pressure point, (upper part of the hip) is related to the functioning of the nerves in the upper buttocks, the lower abdomen, the hips, the sacrum, and the legs.

6. Regulating the operation of the ductless endocrine glands

The endocrine glands, ductless glands that secrete their products directly into the blood stream, are responsible for chemical balance and the harmonious interaction of all of the organs that make up the living human body. The products secreted by these glands are called hormones. The hormones produced by these glands are secreted in minute amounts, which are, however, sufficient to have improtant effects on all the body systems. The endocrine glands include the following: the pituitary gland (three lobes), pineal body thyroid gland, parathyroid glands, thymus gland, pancreas, adrenal gland, testicles, and ovaries. Shiatsu pressure can help regulate the operation of these glands.

7. Stimulating the normal functioning of the internal organs

Shiatsu pressure on the shoulder blades, back, and abdomen helps ensure that the internal organs function as they must to nourish the body properly, oxygenate the blood, and remove waste products regularly and smoothly.

Chapter 2 | Shiatsu Techniques

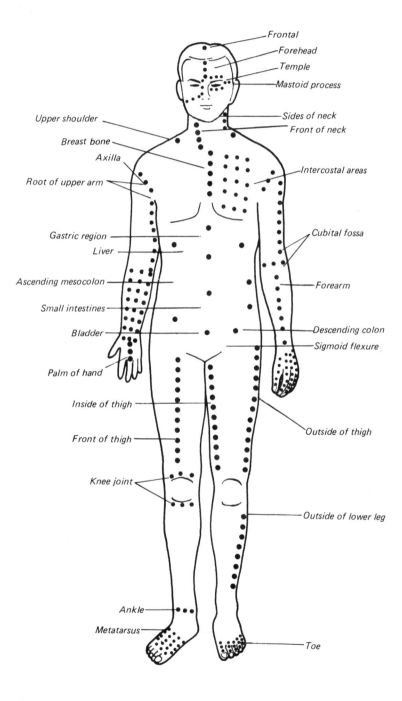

Frontal

Forehead

Temple

Mastoid process

Upper shoulder

Sides of neck

Front of neck

Breast bone

Axilla

Root of upper arm

Intercostal areas

Gastric region

Cubital fossa

Liver

Ascending mesocolon

Forearm

Small intestines

Bladder

Descending colon

Sigmoid flexure

Palm of hand

Inside of thigh

Front of thigh

Outside of thigh

Knee joint

Outside of lower leg

Ankle

Metatarsus

Toe

Hand Movements

Proʋaʋly no tool or implement in the world is capable of as great variety and subtlety of movement and action as the human hand, which begins to move even during the fetal stage of the infant. The fingers are equipped with a number of highly sensitive tactile and thermal receptors located in the tips, or balls, the zones bearing the characteristic patterns of lines and whorls that make fingerprints. The Meissner tactile corpuscles, or touch receptors, give sense data on tactile stimuli. The Pacinian corpuscles, or deep-pressure receptors, provide sense data on pressures and their intensities (Fig. 1). The Krause corpuscles provide information sensations of cold, and the Ruffini corpuscles give data on warm sensations. Nerve endings are distributed throughout this region to carry sense data to the brain, which immediately issues commands for action gauged to the sensation and its intensity.

Fig. 1. Skin covering the balls of the human fingers is without hair follicles.

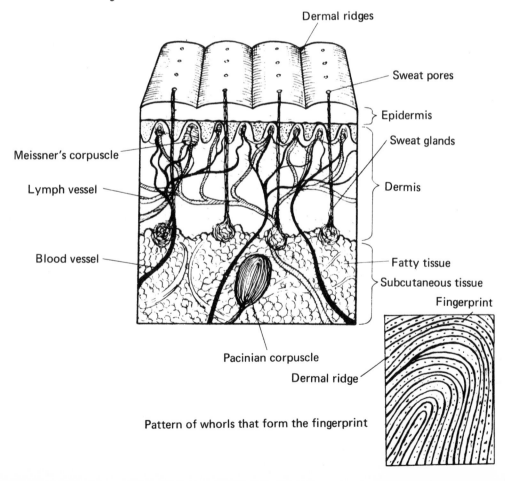

Pattern of whorls that form the fingerprint

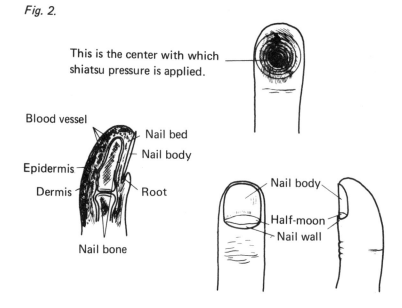

Fig. 2.

This is the center with which shiatsu pressure is applied.

Blood vessel

Nail bed

Nail body

Epidermis

Dermis

Root

Nail bone

Nail body

Half-moon

Nail wall

Shiatsu is concerned with the use of the palms, fingers, and thumbs. There are two natural kinds of thumb. The so-called *amate* (or gentle thumb) is naturally curved and soft. The so-called *nigate* (or hard thumb) is hard and straight. The former is gentle and pleasing, but it lacks sufficient strength to deal with cases of chronic stiffness or paralysis, which require the hard thumb. Through years of training, the shiatsu practitioner learns to put the natural qualities of his fingers to best use and gradually develops the resilience and sensitivity demanded in his work. Furthermore, the sensory receptors in the fingers become remarkably sensitive.

The fingers of the patient provide the shiatsu practitioner with much valuable information because they reflect bodily conditions. If the body is deficient in water or if metabolism is defective, the skin of the fingers will be dry and flaky. When the endocrine glands malfunction, the hands become clammy and excessively moist. The fingernails too reveal the state of health of the patient. For instance, nourishment is probably unbalanced when the half-moons of the nails disappear, when vertical streaks develop, or when the nails break very easily (Fig. 2).

Characteristics of the Thumbs

1. The thumb may be of the soft or hard varieties described in the preceding section.
2. The comparatively great size of the thumb means that it has a wider distribution of sensory receptors and is more sensitive to tactile contacts.
3. The thumb is apposable to the other fingers and has the widest range of movement of all the digits.
4. The thumb consists of only two bones and one joint, whereas the other fingers consist of three bones and two joints.
5. The large, sturdy outermost bone of the thumb has great support strength and permits applications of intense pressure.
6. Repeated shiatsu pressure softens the balls of the thumbs and intensifies their tactile sensitivity.

Shiatsu Methods

Ways of applying speed and degrees of pressure must be varied to suit the part of the body being treated and the condition of the patient.

1. Ordinary shiatsu pressure application

This is the most widely used of all the methods. Apply gentle pressure for from three to five seconds on each point. Gently release (Fig. 3).

Fig. 3. Ordinary shiatsu pressure application

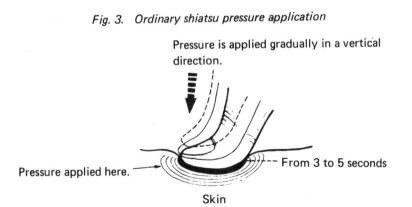

Pressure is applied gradually in a vertical direction.

Pressure applied here.

From 3 to 5 seconds

Skin

2. Repeated easy pressure

Each application of pressure is slightly longer than the ordinary —from five to six seconds. Without removing your fingers from the spot being treated, release pressure. Then gently apply pressure again to the same place. Repeat this process two or three times (Fig. 4).

Fig. 4. Repeated easy pressure

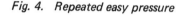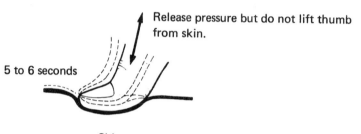

Release pressure but do not lift thumb from skin.

5 to 6 seconds

Skin

Series applications of ordinary pressure

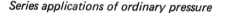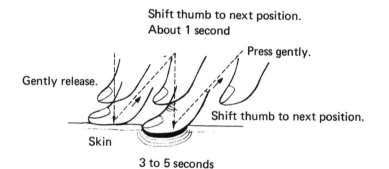

Shift thumb to next position.
About 1 second

Press gently.

Gently release.

Shift thumb to next position.

Skin

3 to 5 seconds

3. Sustained pressure

Pressure is applied for from five to ten seconds in the same place. Applications of such durations are made on the stomach or the eyes with the palms of the hands. In certain cases, sustained pressure is applied with the fingers (Fig. 5).

Fig. 5. Sustained pressure

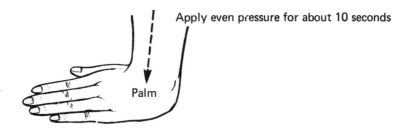

Apply even pressure for about 10 seconds

Palm

4. Suction pressure

This method requires considerable skill.   Using either the palms or the four fingers, press with a slight roll so that the skin of the part being treated is either pushed upward toward your hand (method A) or pulled upward toward your hand (method B). Suction pressure is applied in wave motions to the abdomen or straight down on parts of the skin over internal organs (Fig. 6).

Fig. 6. Suction pressure

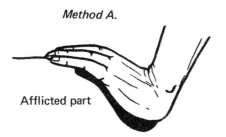

Method A.

Afflicted part

Method B.

The patient's skin must come into close contact with the practitioner's hand, which must press upward.

The patient's skin comes into close contact with the practioner's hand, which pulls forward and upward.
Afflicted part

5. Flowing pressure

Pressure is applied for only one or two seconds in rhythmic repetitions on three points in a horizontal line across the part of the body being treated. This method is very good for treating the shoulder blades (Fig. 7).

Fig. 7. Flowing pressure

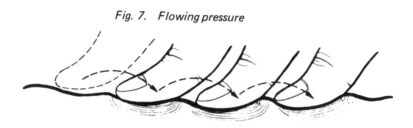

Series of applications with one thumb (1 to 2 seconds)

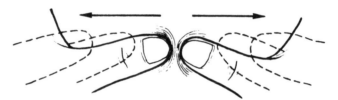

Applications with first one thumb then the other in rapid rhythmical series

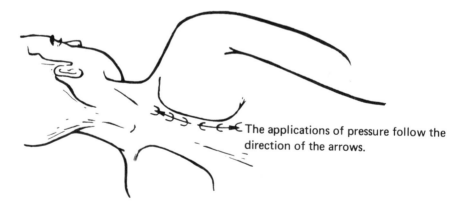

The applications of pressure follow the direction of the arrows.

6. Concentrated pressure

Repeated, concentrated applications of pressure are required to treat parts of the body where the muscles are especially tight. Regulate the duration and degree of pressure according to the condition of the patient (Fig. 8).

Fig. 8. Concentrated pressure

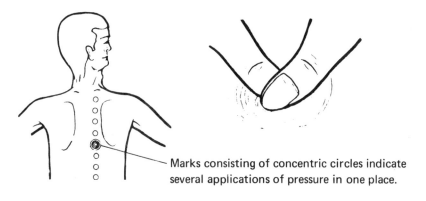

Marks consisting of concentric circles indicate several applications of pressure in one place.

Regulating Shiatsu Pressure

1. Very light

No more than a touch, very light pressure is called for in the treatment of infants or of special, delicate conditions.

2. Light

In dealing with cases in which pressure immediately produces pain, put very little of your body weight on your fingers and press lightly. This kind of pressure application is safe to use with the very young and the very old.

3. Pleasant

This kind of pressure usually produces a pleasant sensation. Even if slight pain is experienced, it is a not unpleasurable pain. Without sharply pressing the fingers, gently lean your weight on your hands and synchronize the pressure with the patient's breathing. This most useful pressure method requires careful control.

4. Strong

Concentrating your weight and strength in your fingertips, press hard, but within the patient's limits of toleration. Even though strong pressure is sometimes applied quickly, it is never sudden or jabbing. Always press gradually.

Rules to Bear in Mind

In practising shiatsu techniques and in using them on patients, always bear the following points in mind.

1. Keep your hands clean and your nails trimmed so that they do not injure the patient or make him uncomfortable.

2. Before beginning to apply pressure, take several deep breaths to calm yourself and promote your own mental concentration and unification.

3. To prevent the development of bad habits, master the shiatsu techniques thoroughly before trying them on a patient.

4. Execute the basic operations in the correct posture. If your posture becomes awkward or irregular, you cannot exert pressure

5. Master the correct basic pressure points. Never apply excess pressure.

6. Apply pressure evenly and rhythmically. This is especially important when you are treating the back.

7. Never press with any part of the hands except the balls of the fingers and thumbs and the palms. Under no circumstances use your elbows or any other joints.

8. Do not have patients suffering from neuritis, stiff shoulders, hernias of the vertebral discs, sprains, or other painful conditions assume awkward or uncomfortable positions. Always observe their motions and be careful to keep them as relaxed as possible.

9. Gauge the treatment duration by the patient's condition and never allow even a full bodily treatment to last for more than from forty to sixty minutes.

10. Throughout the treatment period, concentrate completely on what you are doing.

Use of the Fingers and Thumbs

1. Thumb pressure

Pressure applied with the thumbs is the most important shiatsu treatment. The thumbs may be used singly or together. When used together, they may be held so that their outer edges touch or so that their tips overlap (Figs. 9 & 10). In treating the carotid-artery area and the bodies of young children, use single-thumb pressure. The general treatment employs both thumbs held side by side. For concentrated pressure, use both thumbs held in the overlapping position.

Fig. 9-a.   Pressure with the thumb

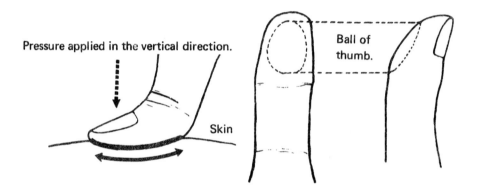

Pressure applied in the vertical direction.

Ball of thumb.

Skin

Fig. 9-b.   Pressure with one thumb

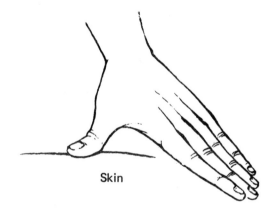

Skin

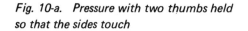

Fig. 10-a. Pressure with two thumbs held so that the sides touch

Fig. 10-b. Pressure with two thumbs held so that the tips touch

Fig. 11. Overlapping thumbs

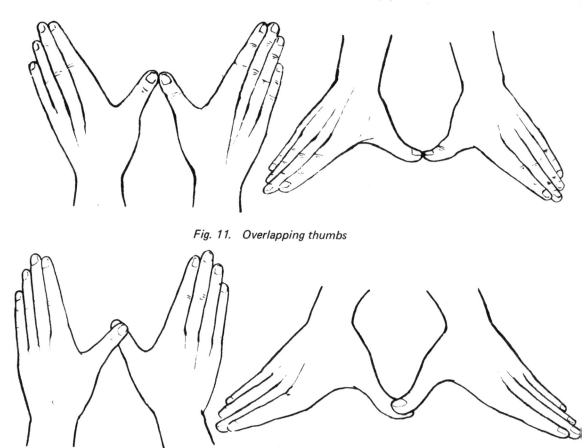

2. Two-finger and three-finger pressure

Use two fingers in applying pressure to such parts of the face as the bridge of the nose. Use it when giving yourself shiatsu treatment to the upper and lower parts of the eyes and the bridge of the nose. In treating a child's back, spread the index and middle fingers wide enough apart to avoid putting pressure on the spinal column. Three-finger pressure is useful in diagnosing the condition of the abdomen and in giving yourself shiatsu treatment to the area of the carotid artery, the temples, the chest, the shoulder blades, and the abdomen (Figs. 12 & 13).

Fig. 12. Two-finger pressure

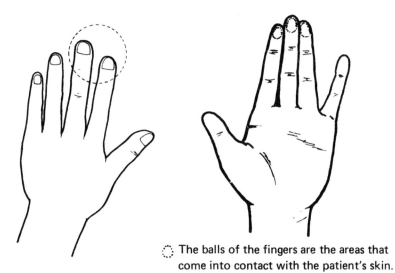

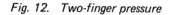

The balls of the fingers are the areas that come into contact with the patient's skin.

Fig. 13. Three-finger pressure

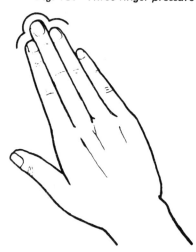

Three fingers used to diagnose a condition

Three fingers used to apply concentrated pressure

3. Palm pressure

Pressure must be applied evenly with the entire palm (Fig. 14). This technique is useful in treating the back of a person who is lying on his side or in giving stroking treatment to a patient's abdomen. Both palms held side by side (Fig. 17) are used in finishing treatment to the back, treating the abdomen, applying vibration pressure, pressing the eyes, or treating the side of the head of a patient in a seated position. Overlapped hands (Figs. 15 & 16) are used in finishing treatment of the back and in giving vibration treatment to the abdomen.

Fig. 14. Palm pressure   *Fig. 16. Pressure applied with crossed palms*

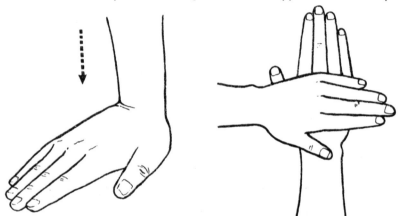

Fig. 15. Overlapping-finger pressure

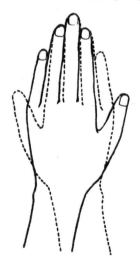

The ball of the middle finger rests on the nail of the index finger.

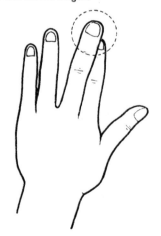

Fig. 17. Pressure applied with both hands;
this is the position used for vibrational
pressure

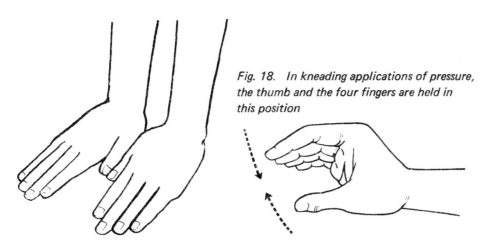

Fig. 18. In kneading applications of pressure,
the thumb and the four fingers are held in
this position

4. Pressure with the thumbs and four fingers

This pressure is applied in a modified squeeze with the thumbs
and the four fingers held in the position shown in Fig. 18.
Fingers and thumbs must exert equal pressure. This method is
employed in treating the side and back of the neck and the calves.

Chapter 3 | Basic Treatment Techniques

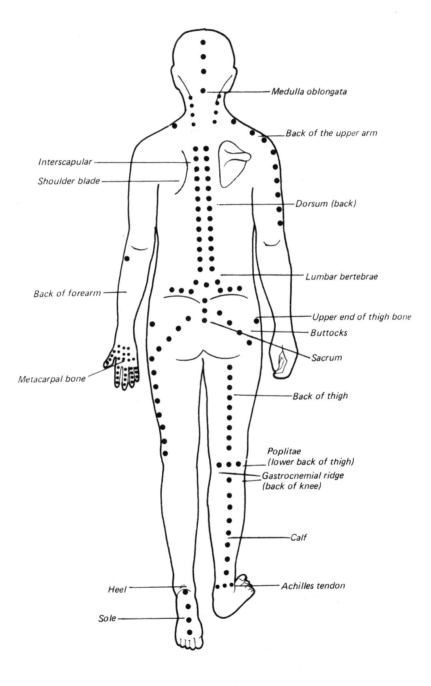

- Medulla oblongata
- Back of the upper arm
- Interscapular
- Shoulder blade
- Dorsum (back)
- Lumbar bertebrae
- Back of forearm
- Upper end of thigh bone
- Buttocks
- Sacrum
- Metacarpal bone
- Back of thigh
- Poplitae (lower back of thigh)
- Gastrocnemial ridge (back of knee)
- Calf
- Heel
- Achilles tendon
- Sole

Patient Lying on His Side

Operation One (Front of the neck)
Patient lies on his right side. Practitioner kneels on his left knee
behind the patient (Fig. 19). He puts his left hand on the floor
in front of the patient. With the thumb of his left hand, the
practitioner presses each of the four points on the front of the
patient's neck (Fig. 20). He repeats this procedure three times,
pressing for about three seconds on each point and applying
moderate pressure.

Fig. 19.

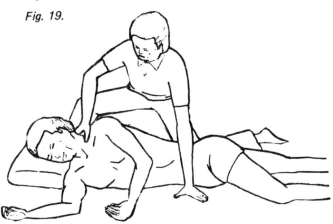

Fig. 20.

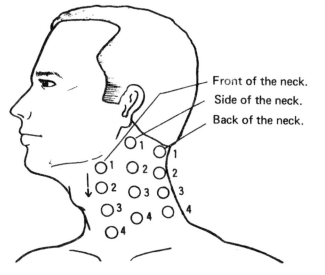

Front of the neck.
Side of the neck.
Back of the neck.

Operation Two (Side of the neck)
With overlapped thumbs (Fig. 21) the practitioner presses each of
the four points on the side of the neck (Fig. 20). He repeats
this procedure three times.

Fig. 21.

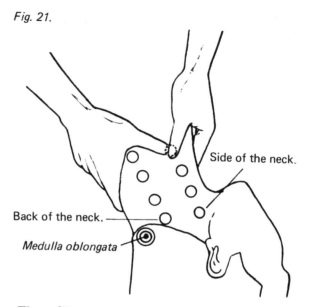

Side of the neck.

Back of the neck.

Medulla oblongata

Operation Three (Base of the neck, medulla oblongata)
Holding the patient's forehead in his left hand, the practitioner
presses on the medulla oblongata with his right thumb (Fig. 22).
Gradually increasing pressure, he presses on this point three times
for about five seconds each time. He must use a slight kneading
motion as he presses. This treatment has a beneficial effect on
the pituitary gland.

Fig. 22.

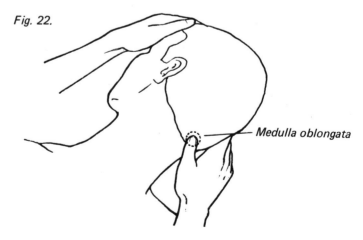

Medulla oblongata

Operation Four (Back of the neck)
Holding his thumbs side by side, the practitioner presses on the
four points on the back of the patient's neck (Fig. 21).
The pressure must be directed toward the center of the patient's
head. The practitioner repeats this procedure three times.

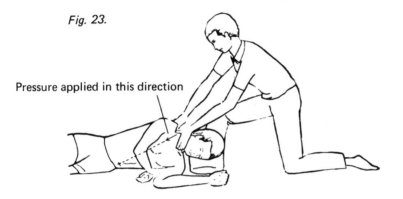

Fig. 23.

Pressure applied in this direction

Operation Five (Upper shoulder)
The practitioner moves to the patient's head and kneels on his
right knee (Fig. 23). With overlapped thumbs he presses three
times on the point on the upper shoulder (Fig. 24).

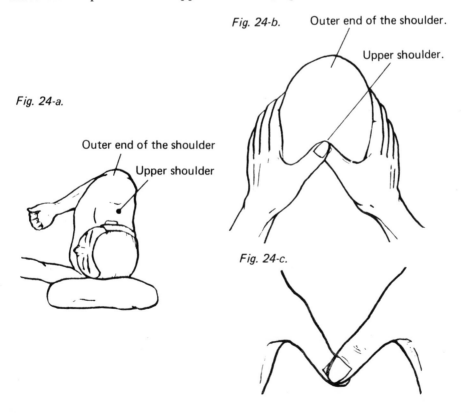

Fig. 24-b.　　　Outer end of the shoulder.

Upper shoulder.

Fig. 24-a.

Outer end of the shoulder

Upper shoulder

Fig. 24-c.

Operation Six (Shoulder blades)
Kneeling upright behind the patient, the practitioner presses three
times on each of the five shoulder-blade points (Figs. 25 & 26).
The thumbs must move in straight, downward, parallel lines
between the inner edges of the shoulder blades and the outer
boundaries of the spinal column. No pressure ought to be applied
on either the shoulder blades or the spinal column.

Fig. 25.

Fig. 26.

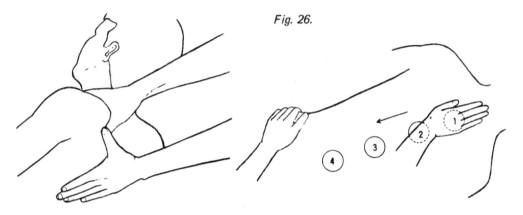

Operation Seven (Back and hip region)
Kneeling on his left knee, the practitioner presses both thumbs on
points 5 through 10 on the back and hip region. He should press
three times on each point. On point 10, he must apply considerable
pressure as he presses three times (Fig. 26).

Fig. 27.

Fig. 28.

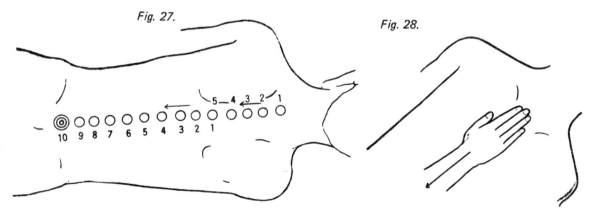

Operation Eight (Downward strokes with the palms on the back)
Placing his left hand lightly on the patient's left hip, the practitioner
applies pressure with his right palm on the four points shown in
Fig. 27. Then, beginning at the patient's right shoulder blade, he
strokes the entire length of the spinal column twice (Fig. 28).
The method is the same when the patient is lying on his left side.

Back of the Body

Operation one (Back of the head)
The practitioner kneels on his right knee to the left of the patient,
who is lying prone with a pillow under his forehead (Fig. 30).
Using overlapped thumbs, the practitioner first applies pressure to
the three points on the back of the head (Fig. 29), three applications
for each point. Caution: When the patient is undergoing treatment
on the back part of his body, he must lie perfectly flat. There
must be no space between his chest and the floor. The only
permissible position for a pillow is under the head, as shown in
the drawing.

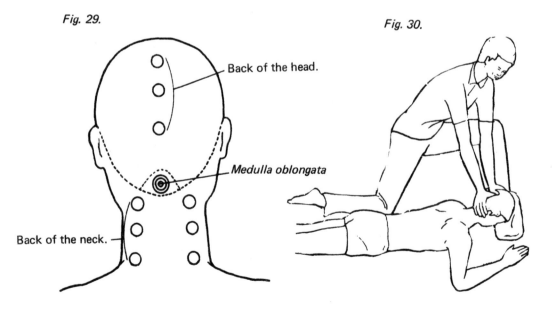

Fig. 29.

Fig. 30.

Back of the head.

Medulla oblongata

Back of the neck.

Operation Two (Medulla oblongata)
With overlapping thumbs, the practitioner presses firmly three times
on the nape of the neck, directing the pressure inward toward
the medulla oblongata (Fig. 29).

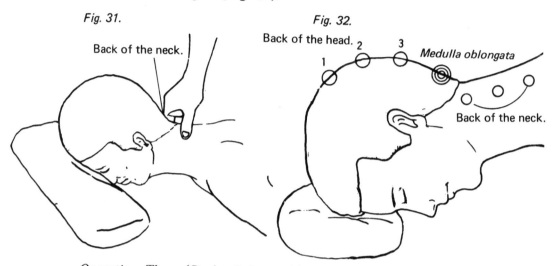

Fig. 31.

Back of the neck.

Fig. 32.

Back of the head.

Medulla oblongata

Back of the neck.

Operation Three (Back of the neck)
The practitioner applies a gripping pressure with the thumbs and
fingers of the right hand to the three points on the back of the
patient's neck (Figs. 31 & 32). Pressure exerted with the fingers
and thumbs must be equal. While doing this, the practitioner
must place his left hand on the front of the patient's head.

Fig. 33.

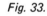

Upper shoulder.

Projection of the seventh cervical vertebra

Fig. 34.

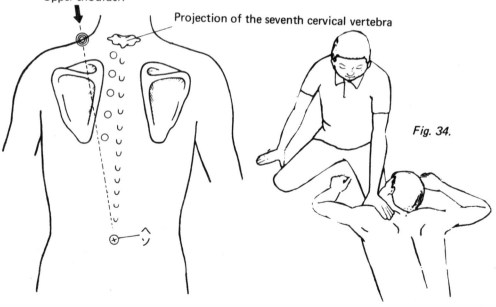

Operation Four (Upper shoulders)
After removing the pillow, the practitioner turns the patient's
head to face to the left. Assuming the position shown (Fig. 34)
in front of the patient's left shoulder, the practitioner presses with
his left thumb on the top of the patient's left shoulder.
The practitioner's thumb must be turned to point toward the
patient's navel (Fig. 33).

Fig. 35.   Fig. 36.

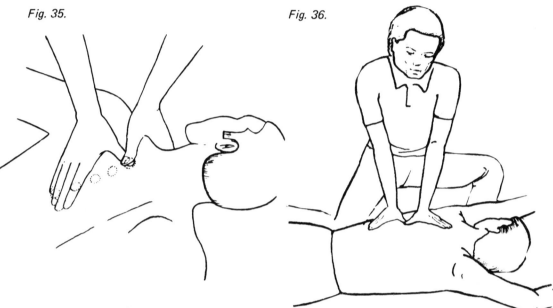

Operation Five (Between the shoulders blades)
Kneeling at the patient's left side as shown (Fig. 35), the practitioner
presses with both thumbs on the five spots located beside and
parallel with the spinal column (Fig. 36). He must press each
point three times, taking care never to press directly on the spinal
column itself.

Operation Six (Lower spinal region and hips)
The practitioner moves the distance of one step back from the
position he occupied in operation five and turns his hands to point
toward the patient's head (Fig. 39). Next he presses each of the
points beside the spinal column from 1 to 10 (Fig. 37). On point
10 he presses hard three times. He then presses three times on
each of the three points above the buttocks. (Fig. 37).

Operation Seven (Sacral region and buttocks)
The practitioner presses three times on each of the three points on the sacral region. He uses both thumbs to apply pressure. Then he presses three times on each of the four points across the heavy muscles of the buttock. (Fig. 37).

Fig. 37.

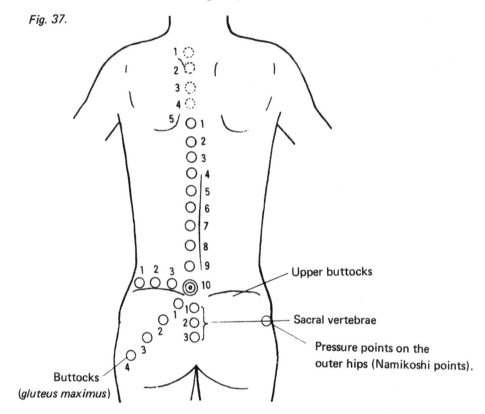

Upper buttocks

Sacral vertebrae

Pressure points on the outer hips (Namikoshi points).

Buttocks
(*gluteus maximus*)

Fig. 38.

Fig. 39.

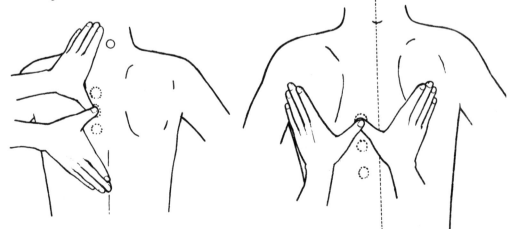

Operation Eight (Namikoshi point)
The practitioner kneels upright beside the patient. With overlapped thumbs, he presses on the Namikoshi point, located slightly above the pelvic joint (Figs. 40 & 41).

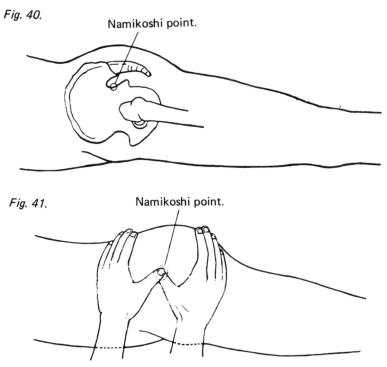

Fig. 40.

Namikoshi point.

Fig. 41.   Namikoshi point.

Operation Nine (The backs of the thighs)
The practitioner kneels on his right knee beside the patient. He presses three times on the first point on the back of the thighs (Fig. 42). This point is located immediately below the crease of the buttock. Pressure applied is strong. He then continues to press on each of the points three times on the straight line running down the thigh from the buttock to the back of the knee (Fig. 42).

Operation Ten (Back of the knee)
The practitioner presses each of the three points behind the knee, beginning on the outermost point and working inward (Fig. 42).

Operation Eleven (Calf and back of lower leg)
Beginning immediately behind the middle of the three points
behind the knee, the practitioner presses each of the eight points
between the knee and the heel. These points are located on a
straight line down the calf (Fig. 42).

Fig. 42.

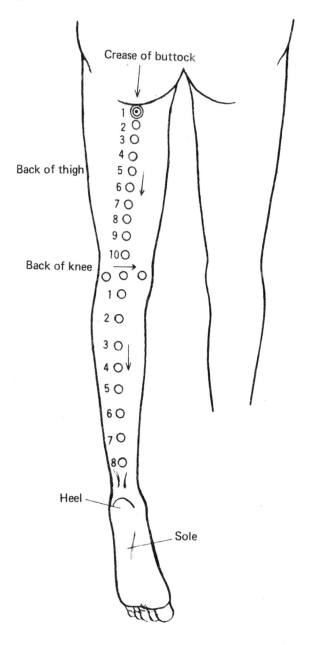

Operation Twelve (Thick of the calf)
The practitioner kneels so that he faces the patient's calf. Taking care to hold his hands as shown in the accompanying drawing, he presses three times on each of the six points on the side of the calf and leg. (Figs. 43 & 44). He must not bend his four fingers as shown in Fig. 43-b, but must bend them back as shown in Fig. 43 on the right.

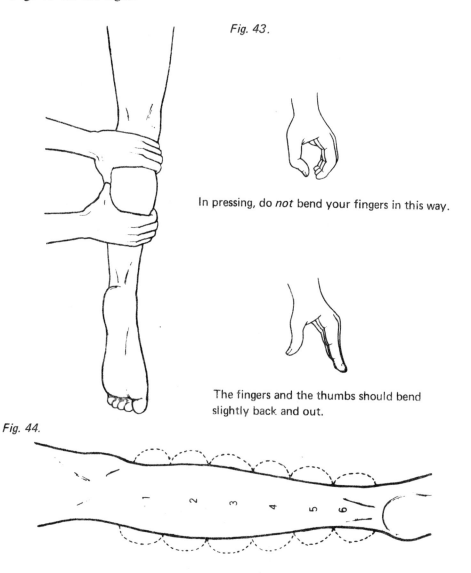

Fig. 43.

In pressing, do *not* bend your fingers in this way.

The fingers and the thumbs should bend slightly back and out.

Fig. 44.

Operation Thirteen (Heel)

The practitioner kneels upright at the patient's ankles. He then presses with both thumbs in the direction of the arrow (Figs. 45 & 46). This pressure extends the Achilles' tendon. He must press this way three times (Figs. 45 & 46). He must then press upward three times on the bottom of the heel as shown in Figs. 47 and 48.

Fig. 45.

Fig. 46.

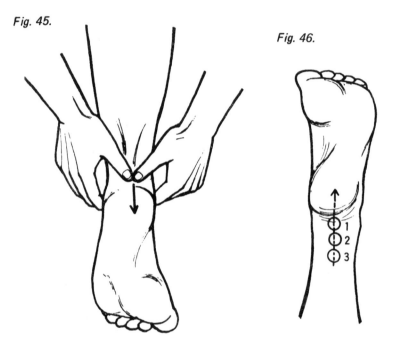

Fig. 47.

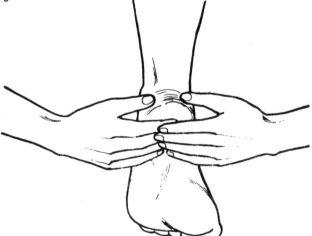

Operation Fourteen (Soles of the feet)

The practitioner kneels on his left knee at the patient's ankles. Beginning with point 1 nearest the bases of the toes, he presses each of the four points three times (Fig. 49). Extra pressure must be used in the three presses given to the arch.

All of the operations described to this point have been concerned with one side of the body. Repeat them all on the other side and finish up with a palm rub of the spinal column (see p. 38).

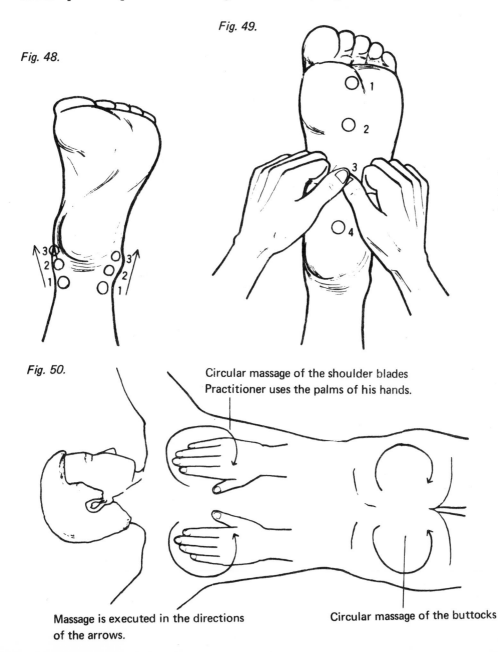

Fig. 48.

Fig. 49.

Fig. 50.

Circular massage of the shoulder blades
Practitioner uses the palms of his hands.

Massage is executed in the directions of the arrows.

Circular massage of the buttocks

Spinal Column (Finishing the back massage)

Operation One (Circular massage of the shoulder blades)
The practitioner kneels on his left knee at the left side of the
patient and with both hands on the patient's shoulder blades,
rubs three times with both hands simultaneously. He must rub
in such a way that the shoulder-blade bones press well into his
palms (Fig. 50).

Operation Two (Up-and-down movement of the side muscles)
The practitioner remains in the posture for the preceding operation,
though he moves away from the patient about the distance of one
step. Placing his hands on the patient's sides (Fig. 51), he slides
them first up then down ten times.

Fig. 51.   *Fig. 52.*

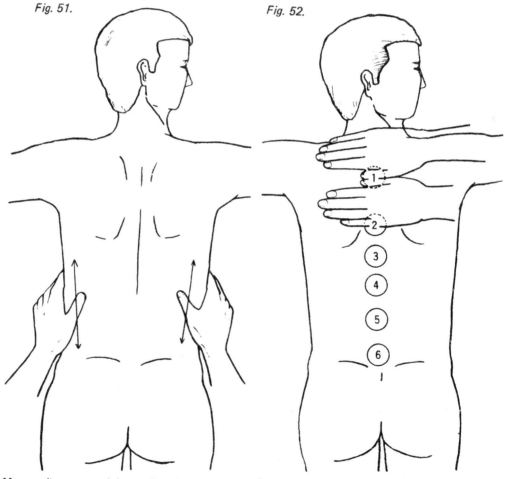

Massage in an up-and-down direction on the
sides of the trunk

Correcting irregularities in the lateral projections
of the vertebrae

Operation Three (Circular massage of the buttocks)
Moving back about the distance of one step from the patient, but
maintaining the posture used for operation two, the practitioner
rubs the patient's buttocks in a circular motion with the palm of
each hand. He first rubs the right buttock three times, then the
left buttock three times, and finally the left and right buttocks
simultaneously (Fig. 50).

Operation Four (Palm pressure on the spinal column)
After kneeling in an upright position facing the patient's right side,
the practitioner raises his hips slightly. Holding both hands
parallel, as shown in Fig. 52, he presses on each side of the six
spinal points. He must press firmly, but gently in such a way
as to force the patient to exhale.

Operation Five (Palm pressure on the vertebral projections)
Kneeling on his left knee, the practitioner puts both hands, crossed,
as shown in Fig. 53, on the six points for treatment of the
vertebral projections. He presses twice on each point.

Fig. 53.　　　　　　　　　　　Fig. 54.

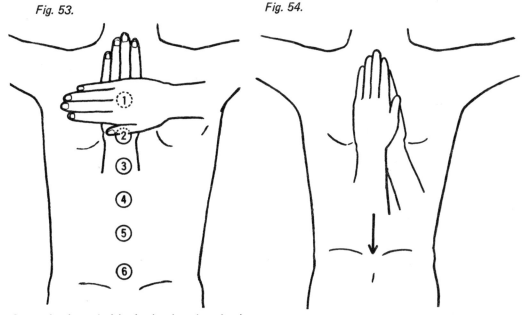

Correcting irregularities in the dorsal projections
of the vertebrae

Stimulating the spinal nerve.

Operation Six (Stimulation of the spinal cord)
Kneeling on his left knee and placing both hands on the patient's back, one on the other as shown in Fig. 54, the practitioner strokes the back bone in the direction of the arrow from the thoracic vertebrae to the sacral vertebrae. He repeats this stimulation of the spinal cord three times.

Patient Lying on His Back

Operation One (Groin)
The patient is lying on his back. The practitioner kneels on his left knee at the patient's left side. Placing his left hand on the patient's left thigh, he makes three gradual, gentle applications of pressure with the palm of his right hand on the patient's groin (Figs. 55 and 56).

Fig. 55.

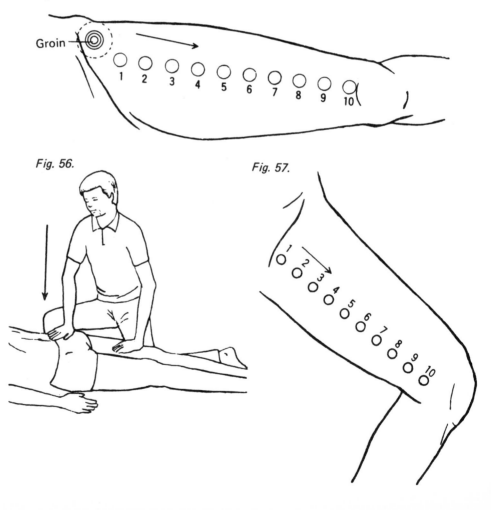

Groin

Fig. 56.

Fig. 57.

Operation Two (Front of the thigh)
With both thumbs, the practitioner presses three times on each of
the ten points from the base of the patient's thigh to his knee
(Fig. 55).

Operation Three (Inner side of the thigh)
Remaining in the position for operation two, the practitioner bends
the patient's leg and with both thumbs presses three times on
each of the ten points from the groin to the knee (Fig. 57).

Operation Four (Outer side of the thigh)
The practitioner kneels upright facing the patient's thigh (Fig. 58-a).
Using both thumbs (Figs. 58-a/c), he presses each of the ten points
from the pelvic joint to a place immediately above the knee joint
(Fig. 59).

Fig. 58-a.

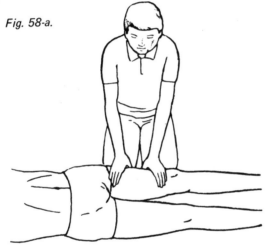

Fig. 58-b.

Fig. 58-c.

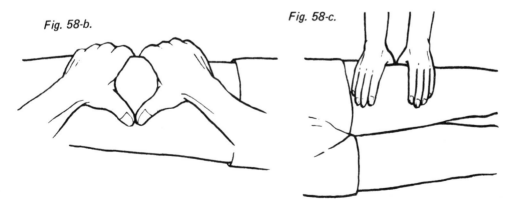

Fig. 59.

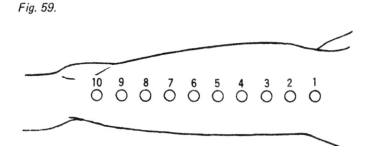

Operation Five (Area of the knee joint)
The points for shiatsu treatment of the knee lie around the
kneecap. The practitioner first presses on the left side from bottom
point to the top point then on the right side from bottom point to
the top point. Nexts he presses alternately right then left points,
three time on each (Fig. 60). He must apply pressure directly to
the kneecap.

Fig. 60.

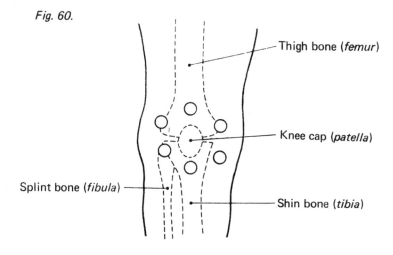

Pressure is applied on the spots marked with a circle.

Operation Six (Shin)
The practitioner kneels facing the patient's shin. With overlapping
thumbs, he first presses three times on a point traditionally called
the *sanri* point (Fig. 61). Shiatsu on this point can be painful;
the practitioner must press neither too long nor too hard. Gripping
the flesh with thumbs and fingers, he then presses three times
each on the six points from the *sanri* point to the ankle (Fig. 61).

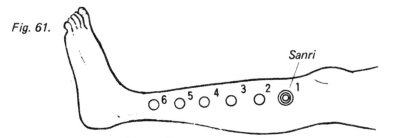

Fig. 61.

Sanri

O⁶ O⁵ O⁴ O³ O² ◎¹

Operation Seven (Ankle)

The practitioner kneels facing the patient's toes, Holding the patient's foot by the toes in his left hand, he uses the thumb of his right hand to press on the three ankle points (Fig. 62). He presses in numerical order; that is, moving from the outer side of the ankle to the inner side.

Operation Eight (Instep)

Remaining in the posture for operation seven, the practitioner supports the patient's foot with his left hand and presses with his right thumb on the four sets of four points each shown in Fig. 62. He presses all of the points one, then all of the points two, and so on toward the ankle. Each point is pressed once.

Fig. 62

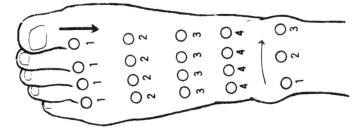

Operation Nine (Toes)

The practitioner holds the patient's ankle in his right hand. Beginning with the outermost joint of the big toe, he simultaneously presses from the top and pulls each of the three joints on each toe, finishing with the little toe (Fig. 63).

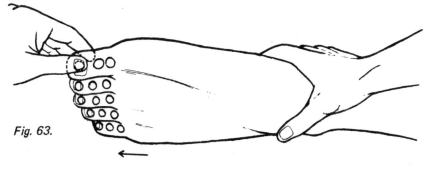

Fig. 63.

Operation Ten (Forward and backward movement of the toes)
Holding the patient's ankle in his right hand, the practitioner wraps
the fingers of his left hand around the patient's toes (Fig. 64).
He then makes the joints of the toes move rapidly backward and
forward ten times. Next he limbers the Achilles' tendon by
holding the ankle in his right hand and raising the foot and pressing
on the sole (Fig. 65).

Fig. 64.

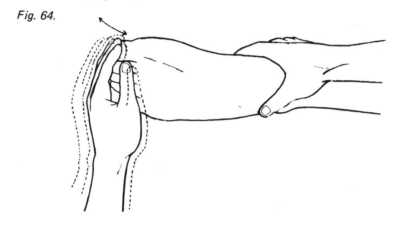

Fig. 65.

Fig. 66.

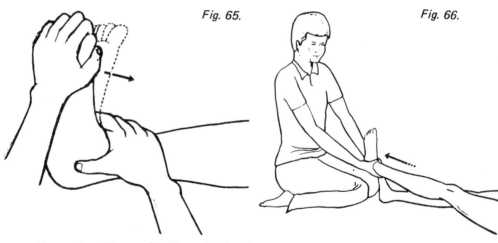

Operation Eleven (Pulling the legs)
The practitioner kneels upright at the patient's feet (Fig. 66).
He places the sole of the patient's right foot against his own left
kneecap. Then, holding the patient's left ankle in both hands,
he raises the patient's left foot about thirty centimeters off the
floor and, gently pulling, lowers it again. The process requires
about five seconds.

Operation Twelve (Inner side of the upper arm)
The practitioner kneels upright facing the patient's armpit (Fig. 67).
With overlapped thumbs, he presses on the point in the armpit
and on the points along the inner side of the upper arm.
He presses each point three times five seconds for each application
(Figs. 68–70).

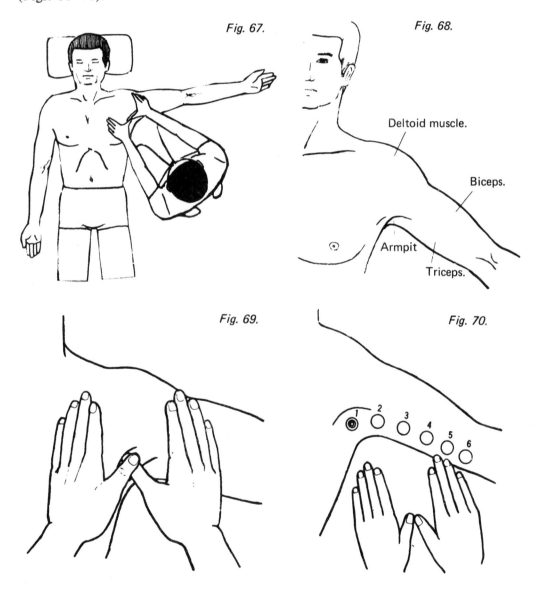

Fig. 67.

Fig. 68.

Deltoid muscle.

Biceps.

Armpit

Triceps.

Fig. 69.

Fig. 70.

Operation Thirteen (Inner side of the elbow)
Remaining in the same kneeling posture but removed from the
patient by about the distance of one step, the practitioner turns
the patient's arm so that the palm of the hand lies up and the
hand is between his own knees (Fig. 71). The then presses with
both thumbs on the three points on the inner side of the elbow.

Fig. 71.

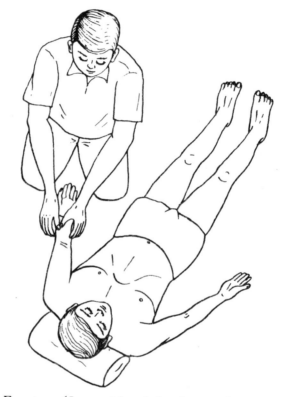

Operation Fourteen (Inner side of the forearm)
Remaining in the position for operation thirteen but placing his
thumbs side by side (Fig. 71), the practitioner presses once on
each of the points on the inner side of the forearm. These points
are arranged in three ranks of nine points each extending from
the elbow to the wrist. In this operation, the practitioner presses
only the first eight points in each rank (Figs. 71 & 72). Before
continuing to the next operation, the practitioner must turn the
patient's hand palm down.

Fig. 72.

Fig. 72.

Elbow   Base of thumb

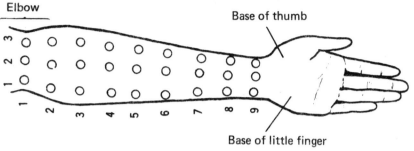

Base of little finger

Operation Fifteen (Armpit, inner side of forearm)
The practitioner kneels at the tip of the patient's right shoulder.
Raising his own hips slightly, he slides the four fingers of his
right hand between the patient's shoulder and the pillow (Fig. 74)
and the four fingers of his left hand into the patient's armpit.
There are three pressure points along the groove of the insertion
of the triceps muscle leading from the collarbone to the armpit
(Fig. 73). The practitioner presses each of these three times with
overlapped thumbs.

Fig. 73.

Groove between the greater pectoral muscle
and the deltoid muscle

Fig. 74.

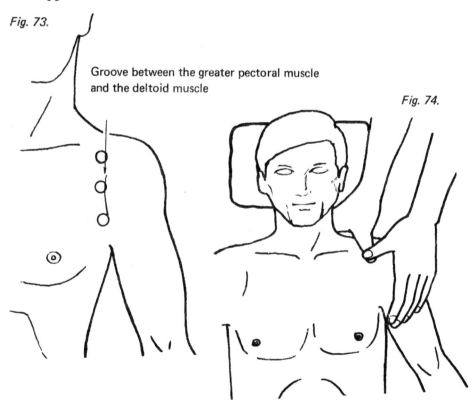

Operation Sixteen (Outer side of the upper arm)
Kneeling upright and facing the outer side of the patient's upper arm, the practitioner uses both thumbs together to press the six points running from the triceps muscles to the elbow (Fig. 75).

Fig. 75.

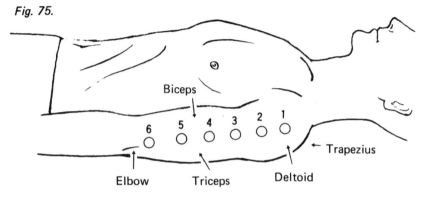

Operation Seventeen (Outer side of the forearm)
The practitioner returns to the posture for operation thirteen (see p. 62). Placing the patient's hand on his own knees, the practitioner uses both thumbs to press the arm *sanri* point (Fig. 76) three times. Still using both thumbs, he then presses each of the eight points from the elbow to the wrist three times. Since the *sanri* point can be painful if pressed too hard or too long, the practitioner must exercise caution.

Fig. 76.

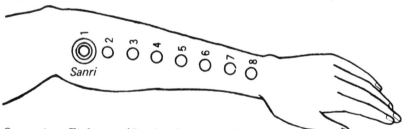

Operation Eighteen (Back of the hand)
The practitioner holds the patient's left wrist in his right hand. Using his thumb, he presses on the points on the back of the hand. These are arranged in four series of three points each (Fig. 77). The practitioner must press each series in numerical order, one application of pressure for each point. He must use his left thumb for the first two series and his right thumb for the next two.

Operation Nineteen (Finger joints)

Holding the patient's left wrist in his right hand, the practitioner presses with his thumb against each series of points on the fingers. The thumb has three series of three points each. Each of the fingers has three series of four points each (Fig. 77). The central series must be pressed independently, but the outer and inner series on each digit must be pressed simultaneously. The practitioner uses his left thumb to press the thumb, index, and middle fingers and his right thumb to press the fourth and little fingers.

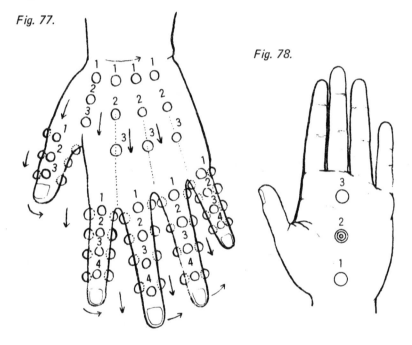

Fig. 77.

Fig. 78.

Operation Twenty (Palm)

With overlapping thumbs, the practitioner presses three times on each of the three points on the palm (Fig. 78). Finally, with overlapping thumbs, the practitioner presses firmly three times on point two in each palm (Fig. 78).

Operation Twenty-one (Arm lift and pull)
The patient raises his hands and arms. Holding both of the
patient's wrists, the practitioner stands, moves to the patient's
head, and raises the patient's hands till they are at about a forty-
five-degree angle from the floor over his head. Holding the patient's
right wrist in his right hand, the practitioner pulls it well to the
patient's ear. He then raises the patient's arm until it is
perpendicular to the floor and immediately releases it so that it
falls toward the patient's hips (Fig. 79). The practitioner must not
force people with stiff shoulders or injuries of the joints to raise
their arms and hands in this way.

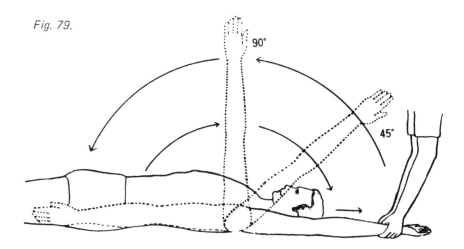

Fig. 79.

Head

Posture
The patient is lying on his back. The practitioner is kneeling
upright and facing the top of the patient's head (Fig. 80). The
practitioner has his kneecaps against the pillow on which the
patient's head rests and holds his hands on his own thighs.
Remaining in this position, he takes several deep breaths to calm
himself and to promote concentration.

Fig. 80.

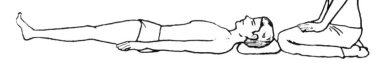

Operation One

The practitioner brings the sides of his thumbs together and holds his hands so that they form a large **W**. With his thumbs, he presses three times on each of the six points running from the patient's hairline down the center of the skull (Fig. 82).

Fig. 81.

Fig. 82.

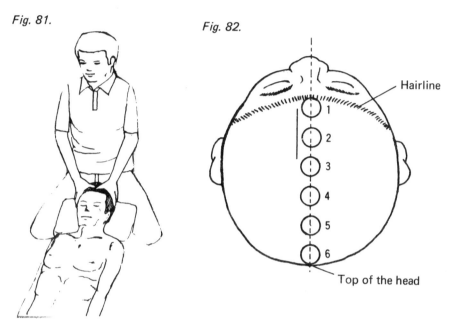

Operation Two

Placing his right hand lightly on the top of the right side of the patient's head, the practitioner uses his left thumb to press once on each of the six rows of points leading leftward from the central line of the skull (Fig. 83).

Fig. 83.

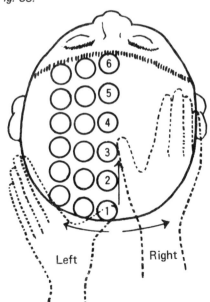

Operation Three
This is the reverse of the procedure in operation two. The practitioner places his left hand lightly on the top of the patient's head and uses his right thumb to press once on each of the points in the six rows of points leading to the right from the center of the skull (Fig. 83).

Operation Four
The practitioner repeats operation one, pressing only once on each point (Fig. 82).

Operation Five
The practitioner repeats operations two and three at the same time; that is, he uses his left and right thumbs to press on each of the three points in the six rows of points leading left and right from the center of the skull (Figs. 83 & 84).

Fig. 84.

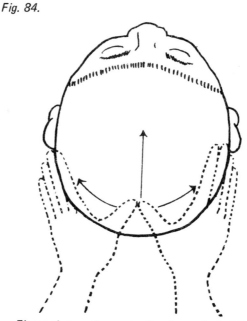

First point on the center line from the hairline.

Operation Six
The practitioner repeats operation one, pressing once on each of the points on the center line. At point six, he presses for about five seconds, gradually increasing then gradually decreasing pressure (Fig. 83).

Facial Region

The posture for this treatment is the same as that used in treating the top of the head.

Operation One
Raising his hips slightly, the practitioner presses three times on each of the three points on the center line of the face between the eyebrows and the hairline (Fig. 85).

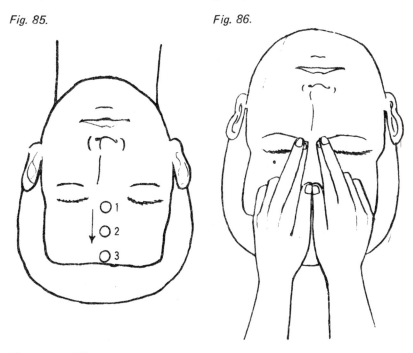

Fig. 85.

Fig. 86.

Operation Two
The practitioner lowers his hips and kneels upright. Placing the tips of the middle fingers over the tips of the index fingers (Fig. 86), the practitioner presses once on each point in the two rows of points running parallel to the bridge of the nose from the inner corners of the eyes to the top of the nostrils. In pressing point three, the practitioner must take care not to close the patient's nostrils (Fig. 87).

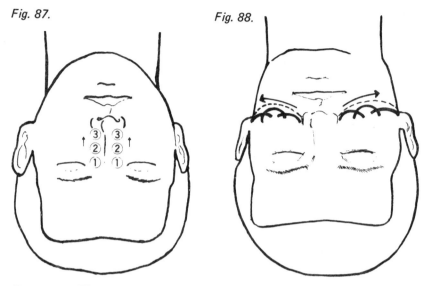

Fig. 87.

Fig. 88.

Operation Three
Using the four fingers of each hand—held close together as in
Fig. 89—the practitioner presses each of the three points on each
of the cheekbones (Fig. 88).

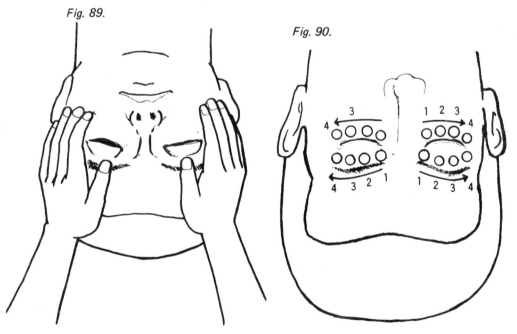

Fig. 89.

Fig. 90.

Operation Four

The practitioner rests his right hand lightly on the patient's forehead. With his left thumb he presses each of the four points on the lower lid of the left eye then each of the four points on the upper lid of the left eye. He presses each point once (Figs. 90 & 91). He must take care not to press directly on the eyeball. He then presses the three points on the left temple (Fig. 92).

Fig. 91.   Fig. 92.

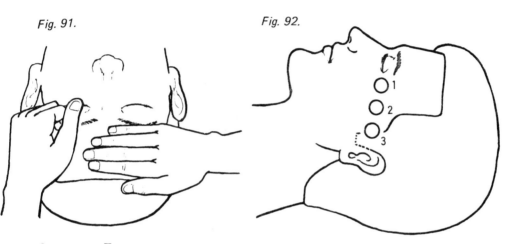

Operation Five

The practitioner repeats operation four on the upper and lower lids of the right eye and on the right temple.

Operation Six

The practitioner lightly rests his hands on the patient's eyes (Fig. 93). He then presses the palms of this hands gently against the eyeballs ten times for a total of about ten seconds. Finally he gently removes his hands. Before resting his hands on the patient's eyes, the practitioner must place a clean cloth or towel over the upper part of the patient's face.

Fig. 93.

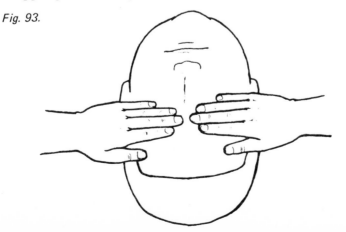

Chest

Operation One
The patient is lying on his back with this legs straight and his hands by his sides. Kneeling upright near the patient's head, the practitioner places his right hand lightly on the patient's chest. With his left thumb, he presses once on each of the four points in the six spaces between ribs on the left side of the chest (Fig. 94).

Fig. 94.

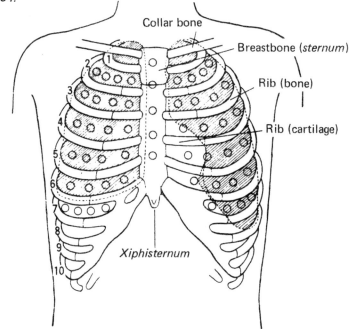

Pressure applied on points marked with a circle

Operation Two
The practitioner repeats operation one on the right side of the body. He must not press directly on the ribs or exert pressure on the lungs (Figs. 94 & 95).

Operation Three
With the tips of his thumbs held together, the practitioner presses each of the five points on the chest bone (Fig. 94). He begins at the collarbone and works downward. He must never press hard or suddenly (Fig. 96).

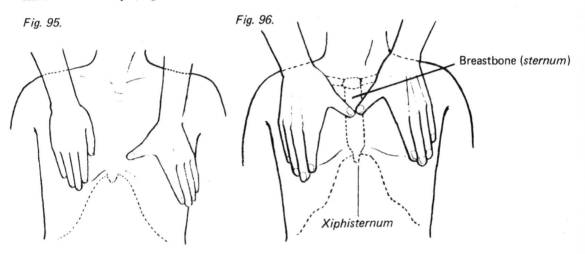

Fig. 95.

Fig. 96.

Breastbone (*sternum*)

Xiphisternum

Operation Four
With both hands, the practitioner rubs both of the patient's breasts stimultaneously in an outward circular motion. He rubs them five times in this way (Fig. 97).

Operation Five
At the conclusion of the five circular massage movements, the practitioner draws his hands upward to a position above the collarbone. He presses the upper part of the chest above the nipples twice in such a way as to cause the patient to exhale (Fig. 98).

Fig. 97.

Fig. 98.

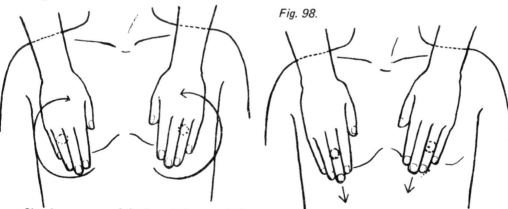

Circular massage of the breasts is executed in the directions of the arrows.

Operation Six
The practitioner draws his hands to the collarbone again, opens his hands so that the fingers point outward, and then gently lifts them from the patient's chest.

Abdomen

Operation one
The patient lies on his back with his legs straight and his hands crossed lightly on his chest (Fig. 99). (This part of his posture has been abbreviated in the diagrams for the sake of clarity.) Kneeling upright at the patient's right side, the practitioner places his left hand on his left knee. With his right palm, he touches the areas above the following organs in the given order: stomach, small intestine, bladder, appendix, liver, spleen, descending colon, and rectum (Figs. 99 & 100).

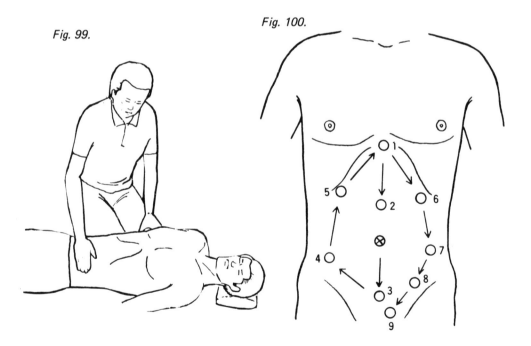

Fig. 99.

Fig. 100.

Operation Two

The practitioner kneels on his right knee as close to the patient's side as possible. Holding his thumbs so that just the tips touch (Figs. 101 & 102), he presses gently on the three points beginning at the sternum and moving to the cartilaginous projection at the bottom of the sternum (the xiphisternum) and to a point immediately above the navel (points 1, 2, and 3 in Fig. 101). He must not exert pressure on the xiphisternum or the navel.

Next he presses on the points (4, 5, and 6 in Fig. 101) between the navel and the pubis. Then he moves up the right side of the patient's abdomen pressing once on point 7, located above the appendix and once on point 8, located above the ascending colon. He then presses three times each on the three points (9, 10, and 11) just below the bottom right rib. He then presses on point 12. Next he moves to the three points (13, 14, and 15) below the bottom left rib; he presses each of these points three times and continues to press the point on the descending colon just below the spleen (points 16, 17, and 18). Finally, he concludes this series of twenty applications of pressure by pressing deeply on points 19 and 20, located diagonally to the center of the bottom from point 1. This series is repeated three times. The practitioner must take care to synchronize his pressure with the breathing of the patient.

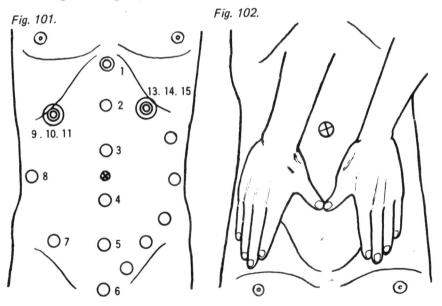

Fig. 101.

Fig. 102.

Operation Three

Holding his thumbs in the position used in the preceding series of twenty points, the practitioner presses three times each on the eight points surrounding the navel (Fig. 103).

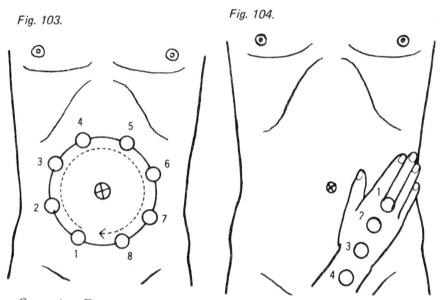

Fig. 103.

Fig. 104.

Operation Four

Kneeling at the patient's right side, the practitioner raises his hips slightly. Placing his left hand lightly on the patient's chest or on his own knee, he uses the palm of his right hand to press the four points from the descending colon to the sigmoid colon (Fig. 104). He presses each point three times.

Operation Five

The practitioner kneels upright at the patient's side and places both palms on the abdomen at the navel (Fig. 105). He then initiates a kind of wave motion by tensing his fingertips so as to pull the ascending colon slightly then by pressing with his palms so as to push the descending colon slightly. He repeats this procedure five times from one side and five times from the other side (Figs. 105 & 106). The pulling with the balls of the four fingers and the pushing with the palms must be done according to the suction method (see p. 29).

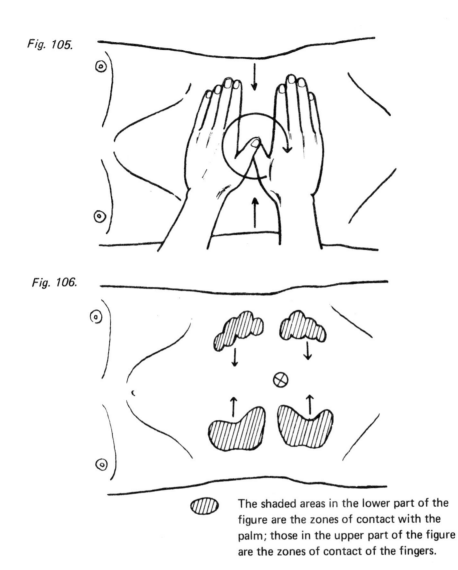

Fig. 105.

Fig. 106.

The shaded areas in the lower part of the figure are the zones of contact with the palm; those in the upper part of the figure are the zones of contact of the fingers.

Operation Six

Placing his palms on the patient's navel region, the practitioner presses deeply and then begins rotating motions (Fig. 105). He repeats this procedure ten times. In this instance, too, he must use the suction method.

Operation Seven
With both palms on the patient's abdomen, the practitioner raises
his hips slightly, tenses his elbows, and makes small vibrational
movements (Fig. 107).

Operation Eight
Kneeling on his right knee, the practitioner places his hands on
the front projections of the ilia (Fig. 108). Pressing first with
the right then with the left hand, he applies pressure to each ilium
ten times.

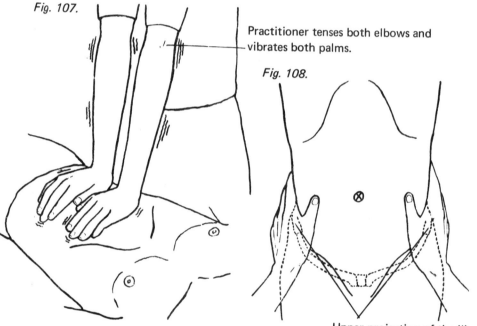

Fig. 107.

Practitioner tenses both elbows and
vibrates both palms.

Fig. 108.

Upper projection of the ilium.

Operation Nine
The practitioner wraps his hands around and under the patient's
waist on a level below the navel (Fig. 109). His fingers must
reach the lumbar vertebrae. Tensing his fingertips, he kneads the
area of the third lumbar vertebra three times. His fingertips must
not come into direct contact with the projections of the vertebrae.
The balls of his fingertips must reach the sides of the regions close
to and beside the third lumbar vertebra. He must bend the tips
of his fingers back slightly.

Operation Ten
First the practitioner raises the patient's trunk with his hands, which are wrapped around his waist (Figs. 109 & 110). He then brings both palms together on the patient's navel and press three times.

Fig. 109. *Fig. 110.*

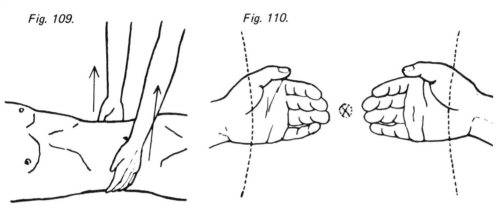

Operation Eleven
With his left hand, the practitioner strokes the abdominal center line from the sternum to the bladder (Fig. 111). Then he strokes the center line with his right hand. He must make ten strokes with each hand.

Operation Twelve
Finally, crossing his hands (right on the bottom) over the patient's navel (Fig. 112), he completes the full course of basic treatment with a vibration massage lasting about ten seconds.

Fig. 111. *Fig. 112.*

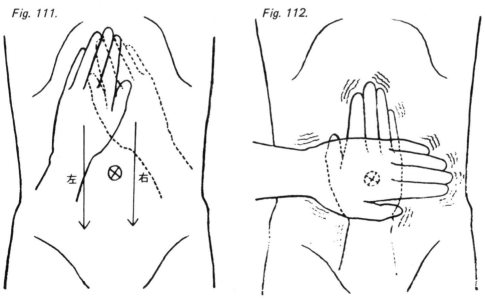

Chapter 4 | Therapeutical Effects

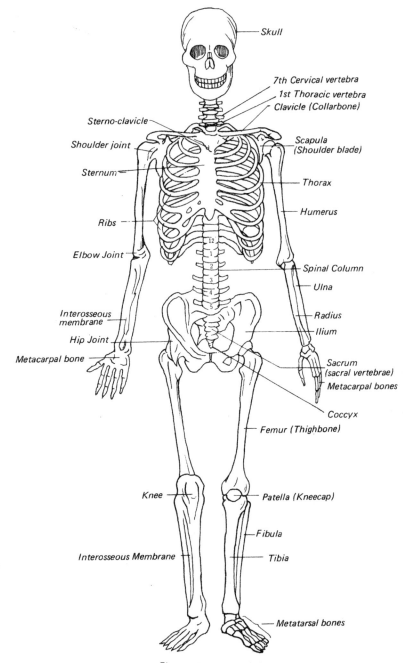

Fig. 22. The human skeleton.

1. Head
Shiatsu treatment of the head can have beneficial effects and
remove the symptoms and causes of the following disorders:
ordinary headaches, migraine, insomnia, cerebral anemia, cerebral
hyperemia, failing memory, neuroses, aphasia, neuralgia of the
back of the head, (cervico-occipital neuralgia), trigeminal neuralgia,
round-spot balding, heaviness in the head, and climacteric disorders.
In addition, it can promote the health of the hair.

2. Eyeballs
Palm pressure on the eyes can temporarily repress the activity of
the heart and slow the pulse because of a reaction in the trigeminal
nerves. But this treatment promotes nervous stability; relieves
eyestrain and crossed eyes; and cures drowsiness, drooping eyelids,
and temporary nearsightedness.

3. Face
This treatment can improve the facial appearance, relieve stuffiness
of the nose, and sinusitis. It can improve the appearance of the
eyes and nose, relieve temporary nearsightedness and eyestrain,
crossed eyes, drooping eyelids, and nervous facial paralysis caused
by the trigeminal nerves. In addition, it can cure tics, toothaches,
and drowsiness and beautify the forehead and the mouth.

4. Front of the Neck
This kind of treatment brings relief from cerebral anemia and
hyperemia, high or low blood pressure, pain in the heart, insomnia,
neuroses, headaches, migraine, toothaches and hiccups. It regulates
the hormone secretion of the thryoid gland, brings relief from the
effects of the so-called whiplash effect occurring in many kinds of
automobile accidents, and helps end hangovers. In addition, it
can help cure climacteric disorders, torticollis, and arteriosclerosis.

5. Side of the Neck
This treatment relieves the discomforts caused by sleeping in

strange positions. In addition, it will cure the ill effects of the whiplash condition, dizziness, ringing in the ears, hardness of hearing, toothache, cerebral hyperemia, motion sickness, hangovers, insomnia, drowsiness, and wryneck.

6. Cerebellum Region

This treatment helps cure insomnia, heart pains, stuffiness of the nose, eyestrain, trigeminal neuralgia, hiccups, sinusitis, whiplash conditions, failing memory, aphasia, drowsiness, nosebleed, vertigo, heaviness and pain in the head, dizziness caused by standing, hangovers, climacteric disorders, and neuralgia.

7. Back of the Neck

This treatment has helpful effects on insomnia, arteriosclerosis, migraine, neuralgia of the back part of the head (cervico-occipital neuralgia), headaches, heaviness of the head, hysteria, failing memory, aphasia, drowsiness, hangovers, climacteric disorders, whiplash condition, and aches of the neck.

8. Upper shoulder

This treatment helps cure stomach pains (shiatsu on the upper part of the left shoulder), pains in the liver (shiatsu on the upper part of the right shoulder), heart troubles (shiatsu on the upper part of the left shoulder), stiffness and aching of the shoulder, numbness in the arms, whiplash condition, neuralgia in the arms, loss of appetite, climacteric disorders, neuroses, and gastroptosis.

9. Interscapular Area

This treatment helps relieve respiratory asthma, pains of the heart (left part of the interscapular area), stomach pains (left part of the interscapular area), liver complaints (right part of the interscapular area), burning sensations in the chest, motion sickness, hiccups, nausea, indigestion, morning sickness, intercostal neuralgia, loss of appetite, palpitations, shortness of breath, lumbago, irregularities of the spinal column, gall stones, and stomach cramps.

10. Back (from the fifth point between the shoulder blades to the tenth point on the hip region)

This treatments helps bring relief from pains in the stomach, intestines, and liver. It provides help in relieving diabetes. In addition, it regulates the secretions of the adrenal hormones, relieves kindey pains, constipation, diarrhea, lumbago, hernias of the intervertebral discs, neuralgia of the ischium, and climacteric disorders. It helps increase sexual potency, cures frigidity in women, stops children from wetting the bed, relieves lumbago, and cures irregular curves in the spinal column.

11. Upper Part of the Buttocks

This treatment brings relief from constipation and diarrhea. It has a reulating effect on the functioning of the intestines and cures chills and menstrual pains. Furthermore, it helps remove fat from the hips.

12. Area of the Sacrum

This treatment increases sexual potency, corrects irregularities in the prostate gland and the bladder, and brings relief from menstrual pains. Furthermore it stimulates the secretion of sex-related hormones and promotes complete erection of the male sex organ.

13. Buttocks

This treatment relieves pains in the ischium, menstrual pains and helps stimulate sexual strength. It brings relief from hemorrhoids, and lumbago. In addition, it helps cure frigidity, stimulates the functioning of the sex organs, regulates the secretion of sex-related hormones, and promotes complete erection of the male sex organ. It stops children from wetting the bed.

14. Area of the Pelvic Joints (Namikoshi point)

This kind of treatment stops diarrhea, relieves hemorrhoids, promotes sexual strength, relieves menstrual pains and menstrual irregularity, cures irregularities in the bladder, stops chills, and relieves neuralgic pains in the ischium. Furthermore it brings relief from hernias of the intervertebral discs, regulates the functioning of the intestines, stops stomach cramps, stimulates the secretion of sex-related hormones, prevents premature ejaculation, promotes complete erection of the male sex organ, and stops children from wetting the bed.

15. Back of the Thighs
This is excellent treatment for pains in the ischium, cramps in the calves, chills, and twists of the knee.

16. Back of the Knes
This treatment brings relief from cramps of the calves, numbness or pain in the legs, gout, aches in the knee, cramps of the soles, swelling of the calves, and twists in the knee.

17. Backs of the Legs and the Achilles' Tendon
This is excellent treatment for cramps or swelling of the calves, numbness, chilling, pains in the heel, twists and sprains of the ankles, and barrenness in women. Furthermore it stretches the Achilles' tendon, cures fevers, and helps remove some of the symptoms of insufficient exercise.

18. Sides of the Heels
This treatment relieves chills, menstrual pains, and fevers and helps stop children from wetting the bed.

19. Soles of the Feet
This kind of shiatsu relieves chills, burning, cramps, and numbness in the feet. It stimulates a reaction that has a regulating effect on the functioning of the internal organs. It relieves swelling and other symptoms of insufficient exercise. In addition, it cures pains in the kidneys, menstrual pains and irregularities, and bed-wetting.

20. Armpits
This treatment relieves neuralgia, numbness and paralysis in the upper arms, stiff shoulders, high blood pressure, and gout.

21. Upper Arms
This treatment relieves neuralgia, numbness and paralysis of the upper arm, paralysis of the medial nerve, gout, and stiff shoulders.

22. Forearms
This treatment helps cure paralysis of the medial nerve, writer's cramp, gout, pains in the heart, and numbness in the fingers.

23. Fingers
This treatment sets up a reaction that helps regulate the functioning of the internal organs and the brain. It relieves writer's cramp, numbness in the fingers, gout, paralysis of the sensory bodies in the fingers, pains in the joints of the fingers, pains in the heart, and inflamation of the tendons in the fingers.

24. Groin
This treatment regulates the operations of the lymph nodes and vessels in the groin, cures frigidity, helps restore sexual powers, relieves chilling, cures barrenness and hernias and promotes a complete erection of the male sex organ.

25. Front of the Thighs
This kind of shiatsu strengthens the stomach and regulates the functioning of the intestines. It relieves ailments of the knee and the symptoms of insufficient walking and exercise. It can also help cure congenital tendencies to easy dislocation of bones.

26. Inner Thighs
This treatment regulates the functioning of the intestines; relieves

sciatica, menstrual pains, and menstrual irregularity; and increases sexual powers.

27. Outer Sides of the Thighs
This treatment is effective in dealing with constipation and diarrhea. It improves the functioning of the intestines and cures beriberi. In addition, it can relieve menstrual pains and irregularities.

28. Knes
This treatment is good for pains in the knee and for rheumatism.

29. Front of the Lower Leg
This treatment is good for chills, swelling, regulation of the functioning of the intestines, menstrual pains, barrenness, loss of appetite, insufficinet exercise, diarrhea, and gout.

30. Ankles
This treatment brings relief from the pain of sprains, from numbness, and from the effects of insufficient exercise.

31. Insteps
This treatment regulates the functioning of the intestines. In addition, it relieves chills, headaches, vertigo, numbness, gout, cramps in the soles of the feet, and the effects of insufficient exercise.

32. Toes
This treatment is good therapy for numbness. It causes a reaction that regulates the functioning of the internal organs. It relieves chills, menstrual pains, frigidity, and the discomfort caused by insufficient exercise.

33. Chest
This treatment has good effects on heart pains, bronchial asthma, intercostal neuralgia, burning sensations in the chest, and insufficient lactation. In addition, it improves the appearance of the breasts in women.

34. Sternum Area
This treatment is good therapy for bronchial asthma, intercostal neuralgia, frigidity, hoarseness.

35. Abdomen
This treatment restores appetite, cures constipation, cures inflammations in the stomach, and brings relief from gastroptosis. In addition, it helps cure stomach cramps, diabetes, ailments of the liver, sciatica, chills, hernia of the intervertebral discs, menstrual irregularities and pains, insomnia, neuralgia, and high and low blood pressure. It cures hiccups, indigestion, frigidity, climacteric disorders, poor digestion, swollen stomach, gout, kidney ailments, barrenness, and gall stones. It helps restore sexual strength, stops bed-wetting, and promotes full erection of the male sex organ.